The

Easy 5-Ingredient

Cookbook

40+ Simple Meal Ideas for Guys with Big Appetites and Limited Time

JOSHUA N. FISHER

Table of content

Contents

Table of content 3

Introduction 8

Cooking Fundamentals for Busy Men 11

Essential Pantry Items 15

Essential Kitchen Equipment 18

Time-Saving Hints & Techniques.......21

Chapter 1 26

Breakfast (5-Ingredient Champions).....26

Eggs Scrambled with Smoked Salmon and Avocado....................................26

Protein Pancakes with Berries and Greek Yogurt....................................27

Breakfast Burrito with Eggs, Sausage, and Cheese 29

Power Oatmeal Bowl with Nuts, Seeds, and Honey.......................................30

Smoothie for Breakfast with Protein Powder, Fruits, and Greens 31

Poached eggs on avocado toast 32

Overnight Blueberry Almond Oatmeal 33

Crepes with Banana Nutella 34

Spinach and Feta Egg Muffins 34

Chapter 2 37

Lunch (Quick and Satisfying) 37

Salad of Steak with Chimichurri Dressing 37

Sandwich with Tuna Salad on Whole Wheat Bread 38

Wrap with chicken Caesar and avocado: 39

Sweet Potato Fries with Black Bean Burgers 40

Soup with leftover vegetables and spices 42

Sandwich with Caprese and Grilled Cheese 43

Salad with Quinoa from the Mediterranean................................44

Tacos with Shrimp con Cilantro Lime Slaw................................45

Salad with Pesto Chicken Pasta.........46

Chapter 3................................48

Dinner (Flavors that are Big and Bold) 48

Lemon Garlic Chicken in One Pan with Roasted Vegetables 48

Chili with Ground Beef and Kidney Beans in 30 Minutes 49

Green Beans and Salmon with Honey-Garlic Glaze 50

Bowl of Korean Beef with Bibimbap Sauce................................51

Primavera Pasta with Shrimp and Fresh Herbs 53

Salmon with Teriyaki Glaze and Broccoli................................54

Skillet Cajun Chicken and Rice 55

Chickpea Curry (Vegan) 56

Grilled Lemon Herb Pork Chops 57

Chapter 4 58

Snacks & Sides (To Get You Through the Day) 58

Chickpeas with Spices & Herbs, Roasted 58

Homemade Tortilla Chips with Guacamole 59

Nachos with Apples, Yogurt, and Granola 60

Energy Bites with Peanut Butter and Banana 61

Eggs Hard-Boiled with Everything Bagel Seasoning 62

Bites of cucumber and hummus 63

Chipotle Mayo Sweet Potato Wedges..64

Fries with Baked Parmesan Zucchini 65

Cinnamon Chips with Fruit Salsa 66

Chapter 5 68

Dessert (Sweet Finishes)....................68

Ice Cream in a Chocolate Mug Cake ..68

Crispy Fruit Salad with Crumble Topping...69

Peanut Butter Cookies 70

Frozen Fruit and Yogurt Protein Shake 71

Clusters of Dark Chocolate with Almond Bark.......................................72

Cups of Strawberry Shortcake...........73

Lemon Blueberry Pudding.................74

Macaroons with Coconut....................75

Bake-Free Energy Bites 76

Bonus Section 78

Weekly Meal Prep Suggestions 78

Grilling Instructions for Meat and Vegetables...79

Spice Cabinet Essentials 79

Leftover Inspirations 80

Conclusion 83

Introduction

It was 7:02 PM, and the usual growl in my gut began. A low growl, at first a whisper, soon rising to a roar. My stomach, a bottomless hole masquerading as human anatomy, demanded food. A sense of sadness swept over me as I looked at my watch. Work had been delayed, and the refrigerator, like my motivation, was nearly empty.

Takeout menus began calling my name, each greasy image a siren song promising instant fulfillment. However, the prospect of another night of manufactured food and empty calories made me feel discouraged. I want a hefty dinner, one that would tame the beast within and fuel my desire for adventure rather than merely sleep.

Then salvation appeared in the guise of a dusty cookbook on the back shelf. "The easy 5-Ingredient Cookbook," as the title suggested, appeared almost too wonderful to be true. Could it hold the solution to my culinary quandary?

I opened the book with a glimmer of optimism and was welcomed by a universe of possibilities. Simple and tasty meals using only five main ingredients. There will be no more trawling the supermarket for unusual spices or spending hours in the kitchen. This was a cookbook for men like me who wanted excellent, satisfying cuisine without all the hoopla.

My stomach growled with anticipation as I glanced over the pages. Spicy chorizo burgers, sizzling beef fajitas, and a filling chicken pot pie - each item promised to satisfy my gastronomic cravings. What's the best part? I just required five materials and a little time.

That night, I set out on a gastronomic adventure with renewed zeal. The perfume of sizzling onions and garlic filled the air in less than an hour, and the growl in my stomach had been replaced by a joyful purr. A surge of happiness came over me as I bit into the first taste of my masterpiece. This was more than simply food; it was a triumph. A win over my time limits, my lack of culinary abilities, and, most importantly, the beast inside.

"The 5-Ingredient Cookbook for Men" became my culinary bible from then on. It gave me the ability to prepare excellent, filling meals that not only satisfied my stomach but also nurtured my spirit. There will be no more takeaway menus or empty fridge sadness. I'd finally figured out how to master the kitchen and satiate my inner glutton.

And now I'd like to welcome you to accompany me on this gastronomic journey. Let's uncover the secrets of simple, yet delectable foods that will satisfy your appetite and leave you feeling energized to take on anything. Welcome to the world of 5-ingredient cuisine, where delectability meets convenience and every meal is a win to be relished. So, put on your apron, gather your five ingredients, and get ready to cook!

Cooking Fundamentals for Busy Men

Let's face it, navigating the kitchen can be a daunting process. Who has time to spend hours slaving over a stove when they're juggling work, errands, and the gym? But don't worry, fellow culinary explorers! This is your passport to deliciousness, created exclusively for busy men who want fantastic cuisine without the effort.

Accept Simplicity

Forget about complicated recipes with obscure components. 5-ingredient magic is your new best buddy. Consider pan-fried lemon-garlic chicken or a robust steak salad with balsamic vinaigrette. The fewer the ingredients, the less time spent on preparation, cooking, and cleanup. Accept the power of simplicity, and your taste senses will be grateful.

Make Friends with Your Freezer

Frozen is not a derogatory term! Pre-cut veggies, frozen meats, and chopped herbs should all be in your freezer. When time is of the essence, this armory of culinary quick fixes will come in handy. In minutes, a bag of frozen stir-fried vegetables and some pre-cooked chicken may be transformed into a delectable supper.

Learn the Secrets of One-Pot Wonders

On hectic weeknights, one-pot dinners are your best friend. Consider soups, stews, risotto, and pasta meals that can be prepared in a single pot, reducing cleaning time. Toss everything in, let it boil, and there you have it! Dinner is ready.

Batch cooking will save you

On the weekend, conquer your kitchen by planning and cooking meals in quantity. Recipes should be doubled or tripled, and individual portions should be frozen for later use. You'll have a supply of ready-made dinners on hand for those times when you're pressed for time.

Accept the Power of Leftovers

Leftovers are not a culinary afterthought; they are a goldmine! Make tacos out of leftover roast chicken, or use leftover chili to make a nourishing soup. Leftovers serve as a blank canvas for culinary innovation, reducing food waste while increasing efficiency.

Don't Be Afraid of the Microwave

The microwave is useful for more than just reheating leftovers. It's a useful tool for preparing quick and healthful meals. In minutes, you can steam vegetables, boil rice or potatoes, or even make a lovely egg omelet. Accept the microwave's convenience and unleash its culinary potential.

Clean as you go

Don't be discouraged by a pile of dishes. Wash and store ingredients as you go to reduce post-dinner mess. A clean kitchen is a happy kitchen, and it will increase your likelihood of cooking again tomorrow.

Keep in mind that practice makes perfect

Cooking is a skill that requires time and effort to master. Don't let your first tries discourage you. Experiment, enjoy yourself, and learn from your errors. The more you cook, the more comfortable you will get in the kitchen.

Most importantly, have fun with it! Cooking should be enjoyable and fulfilling, not work. Celebrate your culinary triumphs, no matter how minor, and share your dishes with family and friends. You'll be whipping up tasty dishes in no time with a little practice and some simple principles, demonstrating that even the busiest man can be a master of the kitchen.

Essential Pantry Items

1. **Finished Goods**
   - Whole wheat flour
   - Oatmeal, rolled
   - Bread crumbs

> Quinoa

> White or brown rice

2. Canned items

> Chickpeas, canned

> Tuna in cans

> Kidney beans, canned

> Diced canned tomatoes

> Hazelnut spread

3. Baking Supplies

> Baking soda

> Baking powder

> Granulated and brown sugar

> Honey

> Cocoa butter

4. Vinegar and oils

> Extra virgin olive oil

> Vegetable or canola oil for cooking

> ACV (apple cider vinegar)

5. Herbs and spices

- Salt
- Chili
- Powdered garlic
- Chilean paprika
- Italian seasoning
- Cumin

6. Sauces and condiments

- Dijon mustard
- Mayonnaise
- Sesame oil
- Teriyaki marinade
- Pesto dressing
- Chipotle mayonnaise

7. Sweeteners

- Sugar

8. Pasta and grains

- Whole wheat grains
- Pasta of your choosing

9. Seeds and nuts

- ➢ Sliced almonds
- ➢ Chia seeds

10. Dairy and Dairy Substitutes

- ➢ Feta feta cheese
- ➢ Greek yoghurt
- ➢ Heavy whipping cream

11. Miscellaneous

- ➢ Lime curd
- ➢ Chocolate pieces
- ➢ Nut butter (Almond butter, peanut butter, etc.)

Essential Kitchen Equipment

1. **Knife for the Chef:** Multipurpose for precision chopping and slicing.
2. **Chopping Board:** Sturdy surface for quick and safe food preparation.

3. **Several mixing bowls:** Various sizes for mixing and preparing ingredients.

4. **Cups and Spoons for Measuring:** Required for accurate ingredient measuring.

5. **Frying Pan or Skillet:** Multipurpose pan for sautéing and frying.

6. **Baking Pan:** An oven-safe baking and roasting tray.

7. **Saucepan:** A medium-sized saucepan for simmering and boiling.

8. **Food Processor or Blender:** To make smoothies, soups, and sauces.

9. **Tongs**: Excellent for food turning and serving.

10. **Spoon made of wood:** Excellent for stirring and blending.

11. **Opener of Cans:** Required for opening canned foods.

12. **Peeler:** Fruit and vegetable peeling that is quick and efficient.

13. **Grater:** To grate cheese, vegetables, or citrus zest.

14. **Colander:** Used for draining spaghetti and washing fruits and vegetables.

15. **Mitts for the Oven:** Required for working with hot pots and pans.

16. **Utensils for cooking (spatulas, ladles, slotted spoons):** A variety of utensils for various kitchen activities.

17. **Set of cutlery:** Additional knives for specialized cutting.

18. **Thermometer for Meat:** Assures correct meat cooking temperatures.

19. **Set of Canisters:** Stores and organizes critical dry commodities.

20. **Spatula:** For delicate item flipping.

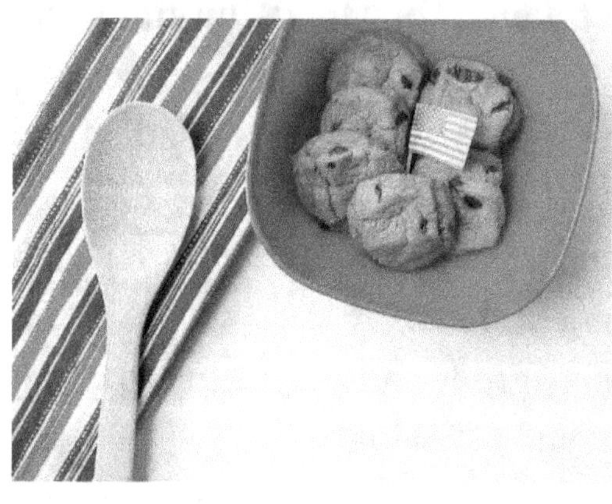

Time-Saving Hints & Techniques

1. Preparation like a pro

Prepare veggies ahead of time: On the weekend, wash, peel, and cut vegetables like onions, peppers, and carrots and store them in airtight containers in the refrigerator. This will save you time all week.

2. Cook in bulk

On the weekend, make double or triple quantities of protein (chicken, beans, tofu) and grains (rice, quinoa, pasta). This way, you'll have ready-made ingredients for the rest of the week.

3. Prepare marinades ahead of time

Marinate your protein while at work or running errands. This will flavor the meat and save you time when preparing dinner.

4. Use pre-cooked ingredients

Keep canned beans, lentils, and pre-cooked chicken or shrimp on hand. You will save time chopping and cooking as a result of this.

5. Using the Microwave

Use the microwave to steam veggies, make rice, or even poach eggs for quick and simple side dishes.

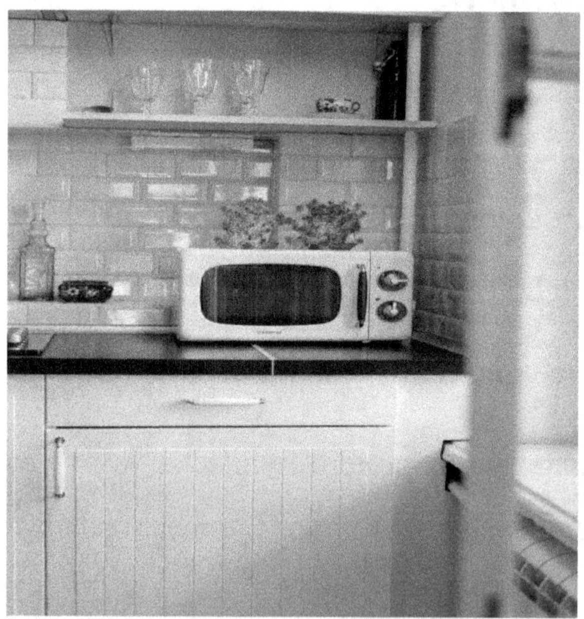

COOKING EFFECTIVENESS:

One-pan meals

For a quick and delectable supper, roast veggies and protein on a single sheet pan.

Multi-cooker magic

Use your slow cooker or Instant Pot to quickly make stews, soups, and curries.

One-pot wonders

For a quick and simple cleanup, cook pasta, rice, or quinoa straight in the sauce.

Simultaneous cooking

Steam your vegetables or cook your protein while your pasta is boiling. You will save time and energy as a result of this.

Reduce cleanup

Line baking sheets and pans with parchment paper to make cleaning easier.

Use foil packages

For a mess-free cooking experience, wrap your protein and veggies in foil packets.

Use disposable containers

For simple cleanup and portion control, cook individual portions in disposable containers.

Clean as you go

To avoid a major mess at the end, wash your dishes while you cook.

ADDITIONAL HINTS

Plan your meals: Make a food list and plan your meals for the week ahead of time to minimize unnecessary shopping excursions.

Frozen veggies are equally as nutritious as fresh vegetables and can save you time cutting and cleaning.

Make use of kitchen tools: A food processor may save you time slicing vegetables, and an immersion blender can assist you in making quick and simple sauces.

Don't be scared to experiment

Don't be hesitant to try new flavors and ingredients. You might be amazed at how tasty a 5-ingredient supper can be.

Keep in mind that the objective is to make cooking quick and pleasurable. You can make tasty and nutritious meals even when you're short on time if you use these time-saving techniques and tactics.

Chapter 1

Breakfast (5-Ingredient Champions)

Eggs Scrambled with Smoked Salmon and Avocado

Ingredients

1. Eggs
2. Salmon smoked
3. Avocado
4. Salt
5. Chili

Instructions

1. In a mixing dish, crack the eggs, season with salt and pepper, and whisk.

2. In a nonstick skillet over medium heat, melt the butter.

3. Pour the whisked eggs into the skillet and gently scramble until barely set.

4. Add smoked salmon and chopped avocado to the eggs, swirling gently to mix.

5. Cook for a further minute until everything is heated through.

6. Serve immediately and enjoy your protein-packed breakfast!

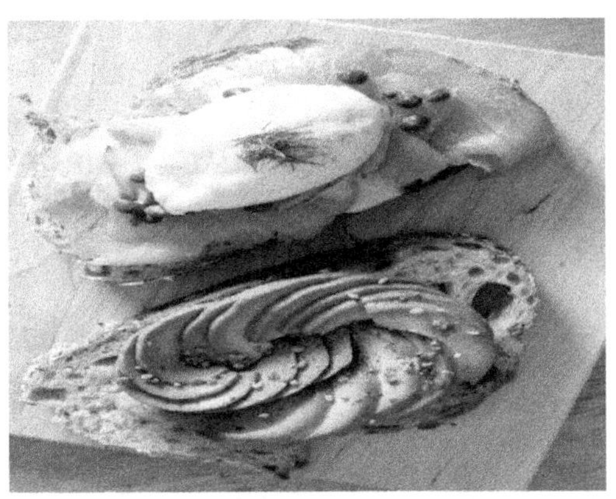

Protein Pancakes with Berries and Greek Yogurt

Ingredients

1. Pancake butter

2. Protein shake

3. Berries in various combinations

4. Greek yoghurt

5. Maple syrup (optional)

Instructions

1. In a mixing bowl, combine the pancake mix and water or milk according to package directions.

2. Mix in the protein powder until thoroughly blended.

3. Pour the pancake batter onto a griddle or pan heated over medium heat.

4. Cook until bubbles form on the surface of each pancake, then flip and cook the other side.

5. Stack the pancakes and top with a dollop of Greek yogurt and mixed berries.

6. If preferred, drizzle with maple syrup and enjoy the goodness!

Breakfast Burrito with Eggs, Sausage, and Cheese

Ingredients

1. Tortillas made from flour

2. Pork sausage

3. Eggs

4. Cheddar

5. Salsa

Instructions

1. In a pan over medium heat, brown the sausage.

2. Scramble the eggs in the same skillet with a pinch of salt.

3. In a different pan or microwave, warm the flour tortillas.

4. Place the cooked sausage and eggs on the tortilla to make the burrito.

5. Season with cheese and salsa to taste.

6. Roll up the tortilla and it's ready to eat!

Power Oatmeal Bowl with Nuts, Seeds, and Honey

Ingredients

1. Oats

2. Nuts (almonds, walnuts, etc.)

3. Seeds (chia seeds, flaxseeds

4. Honey

5. Milk

Instructions

1. Cook oats according to package directions on the stovetop or in the microwave.

2. Top the cooked oats with a nut and seed mixture.

3. Drizzle with honey to taste.

4. To get the correct consistency, add a dash of milk or water.

5. Stir thoroughly and serve for a wholesome and filling breakfast!

Smoothie for Breakfast with Protein Powder, Fruits, and Greens

Ingredients

1. Protein shake

2. Mixed fruits (bananas, berries, etc.)

3. Kale or spinach

4. Greek yoghurt

5. Almond milk

Instruction

1. Combine protein powder, various fruits, spinach or kale, yogurt, and almond milk in a blender.

2. Blend until the mixture is smooth and creamy.

3. If necessary, adjust the consistency by adding additional almond milk.

4. Pour into a glass and enjoy a refreshing and nutritious smoothie to start your day!

Poached eggs on avocado toast

Ingredients

1. Whole wheat bread
2. Avocado
3. Eggs
4. Salt
5. Chili

Instructions

1. Toast the pieces of whole-grain bread.
2. Spread mashed avocado on toasted bread.

3. Place the poached eggs on top of the avocado.

4. Season to taste with salt and pepper.

5. Enjoy a tasty and nutritious breakfast!

Overnight Blueberry Almond Oatmeal

Ingredients

1. Oatmeal, rolled

2. Almond milk

3. Strawberries

4. Sliced almonds

5. Honey

Instructions

1. In a container, combine rolled oats, almond milk, and honey.

2. Blueberries and almond slices are optional.

3. Refrigerate overnight after thoroughly stirring.

4. Give it a nice stir in the morning and enjoy your delicious overnight oats!

Crepes with Banana Nutella

Ingredients

1. Pancakes
2. hazelnut spread
3. chopped nuts
4. Sliced banana
5. Sugar

Instructions

1. On a crepe, spread Nutella.

2. Mix in the banana slices and nuts.

3. Crepes can be folded or rolled.

4. Sprinkle with powdered sugar.

5. Enjoy a delicious banana Nutella crepe!

Spinach and Feta Egg Muffins

Ingredients

1. Eggs
2. Spinach
3. Feta feta cheese
4. Salt
5. Chili

Instructions

1. Preheat the oven to 350°F (180°C).
2. Whisk eggs in a mixing bowl and season with salt and pepper.
3. Mix in the spinach and feta crumbles.
4. Fill muffin cups halfway with the mixture.
5. Bake the eggs for 15-20 minutes, or until they are set.
6. Enjoy a flavorful spinach and feta egg muffin in no time!

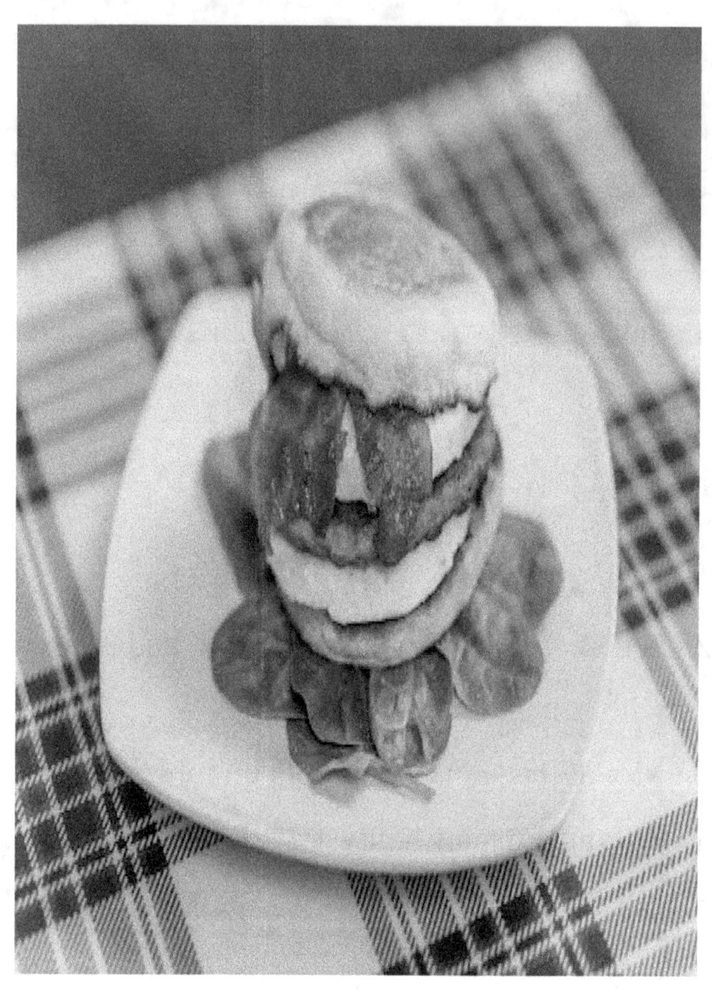

Chapter 2

Lunch (Quick and Satisfying)

Salad of Steak with Chimichurri Dressing

Ingredients

1. Steak

2. Salad greens, mixed

3. Tomatoes, cheery

4. Red onions

Instructions

1. Season the steak with salt and pepper to taste.

2. Grill or pan-sear the steak until done to your liking.

3. Cooked steak should be cut into thin pieces.

4. Salad greens, cherry tomatoes, and sliced red onion should all be combined in a bowl.

5. Drizzle the Chimichurri sauce over the salad and top with the cut meat.

6. Gently toss and serve a tasty steak salad!

Sandwich with Tuna Salad on Whole Wheat Bread

Ingredients

1. Canned tuna

2. Dijon mustard

3. Cauliflower

4. Whole grain bread

5. Spinach

Instructions

1. Place the canned tuna in a mixing basin.

2. To the tuna, add mayonnaise and finely sliced celery.

3. Mix until everything is properly blended.

4. Distribute the tuna mixture on whole wheat bread.

5. To build a sandwich, top with lettuce and another slice of bread.

6. Cut in half and enjoy a fast and delicious tuna salad sandwich!

Wrap with chicken Caesar and avocado:

Ingredients

1. Chicken bread grilled

2. Salad dressing

3. Lettuce Romaine

4. Tortilla made from flour

5. Slices of avocado

Instructions

1. Grill the chicken breast into strips.

2. Toss the chicken strips with the Caesar dressing in a mixing basin.

3. Place a few Romaine lettuce leaves in the center of a flour tortilla.

4. Add the avocado slices and the seasoned chicken pieces.

5. Roll the tortilla into a wrap.

6. Cut the chicken Caesar wrap in half diagonally and enjoy!

Sweet Potato Fries with Black Bean Burgers

Ingredients

1. Black bean burgers (purchased or homemade)

2. Buns for hamburgers

3. Spinach

4. Sliced tomatoes

5. Fries made with sweet potatoes

Instructions

1. Cook the black bean burgers as directed on the packet.
2. If desired, toast the burger buns.
3. Burgers should be topped with lettuce, tomato slices, and a cooked black bean patty.
4. Serve with sweet potato fries for a filling supper.
5. Enjoy a delicious black bean burger with crunchy sweet potato fries!

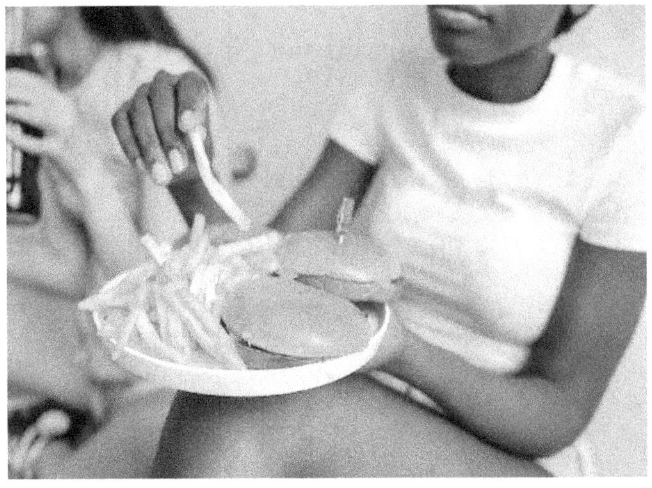

Soup with leftover vegetables and spices

Ingredients

1. Meat leftovers (chicken, beef, or pig)
2. Vegetables (carrots, peas, and corn)
3. Powdered garlic
4. Chicken or veggie broth
5. Italian seasoning

Instructions

1. Make bite-sized chunks of leftover meat.
2. Combine mixed veggies and cut meats in a saucepan.
3. Fill the container halfway with broth.
4. Garlic powder and Italian spice to taste.
5. Simmer until the veggies are soft and the flavors have combined.

6. For a quick and healthy lunch, serve a bowl of leftover soup!

Sandwich with Caprese and Grilled Cheese

Ingredients

1. Bread
2. Cheese, mozzarella
3. Toasted tomatoes
4. Basil
5. Margarine

Instructions

1. Assemble the sandwich by layering it with mozzarella, tomato, and basil.
2. Butter the bread's outside edges.
3. Grill the bread until the cheese is melted and brown.

4. Enjoy a delicious Caprese grilled cheese sandwich!

Salad with Quinoa from the Mediterranean

Ingredients

1. Quinoa
2. Cherry Tomatoes
3. Cucumber
4. Feta feta cheese
5. Extra virgin olive oil

Instructions

1. Follow the package instructions for cooking the quinoa.
2. Combine quinoa, halved cherry tomatoes, chopped cucumber, and crumbled feta in a mixing bowl.
3. Drizzle with olive oil and gently stir.

4. Serve a cool Mediterranean quinoa salad!

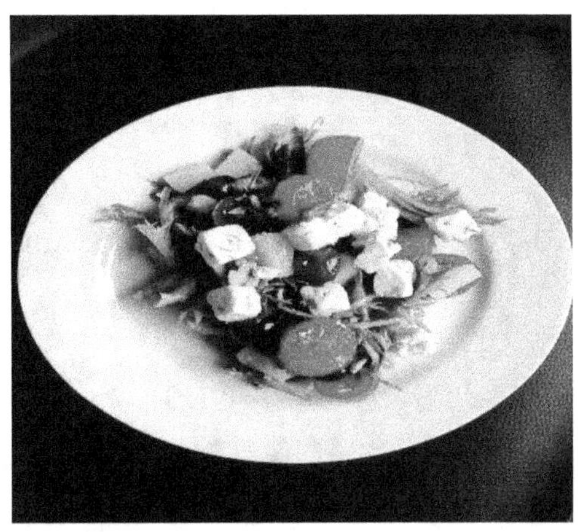

Tacos with Shrimp con Cilantro Lime Slaw

Ingredients

1. Steamed shrimp

2. Tortillas

3. Cauliflower

4. Coriander

5. Lime

Instructions

1. Cook the shrimp until they are pink and opaque.

2. Combine the shredded cabbage, cilantro, and lime juice in a mixing dish.

3. Tacos should be topped with shrimp and salad.

4. If desired, squeeze on more lime.

5. Delicious shrimp tacos with cilantro lime slaw!

Salad with Pesto Chicken Pasta

Ingredients

1. Pasta

2. Grilled chicken

3. Tomatoes

4. Pesto

5. Parmigiano-Reggiano

Instructions

1. Cook the pasta as directed on the packet.

2. Combine the cooked pasta, grilled chicken, halved cherry tomatoes, and pesto in a mixing bowl.

3. Toss thoroughly and serve with Parmesan cheese on top.

4. Serve a refreshing pesto chicken pasta salad!

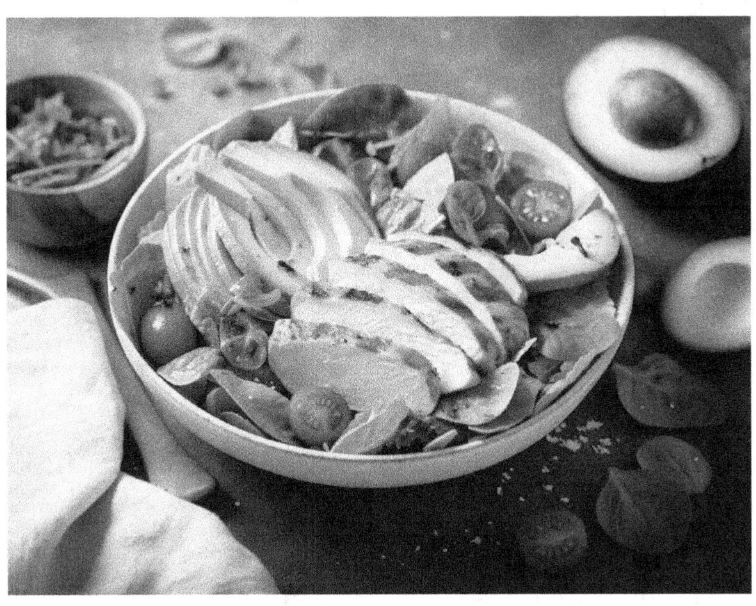

Chapter 3

Dinner (Flavors that are Big and Bold)

Lemon Garlic Chicken in One Pan with Roasted Vegetables

Ingredients

1. Chicken
2. Lemon
3. Cloves of garlic
4. Various veggies (carrots, broccoli, bell peppers etc.)
5. Extra virgin olive oil

Instructions

1. Preheat the oven to 425 °F (220°C).
2. Season the chicken thighs with salt, pepper, and garlic powder.

3. Place the chicken and veggies on a baking sheet.

4. Drizzle with olive oil and sprinkle with lemon juice.

5. Bake for 25-30 minutes, or until the chicken is cooked through and the veggies are soft.

6. With lemony garlic chicken and roasted vegetables, you can make a delightful one-pan supper!

Chili with Ground Beef and Kidney Beans in 30 Minutes

Ingredients

1. Beef ground

2. Canned kidney beans

3. Canned tomatoes

4. Chipotle powder

5. Onion

Instructions

1. In a large saucepan over medium heat, brown the ground beef.

2. Cook until the onions are transparent.

3. Pour in the canned chopped tomatoes and kidney beans.

4. To taste, season with chili powder.

5. Simmer, stirring periodically, for 20-30 minutes.

6. Serve a hearty bowl of chili topped with your favorite toppings!

Green Beans and Salmon with Honey-Garlic Glaze

Ingredients

1. Salmon fillets

2. Honey

3. Cloves of garlic

4. Sesame oil

5. Fresh green beans

Instructions

1. Preheat the oven to 400°F (200°C).

2. Line a baking sheet with parchment paper and place the salmon fillets on it.

3. To make a glaze, combine honey, minced garlic, and soy sauce in a mixing dish.

4. Brush the salmon fillets with the glaze.

5. Arrange the salmon on a bed of fresh green beans.

6. Bake for 12-15 minutes, or until the salmon is done.

7. Serve with soft green beans and a delicious honey-garlic glazed fish!

Bowl of Korean Beef with Bibimbap Sauce

Ingredients

1. Beef ground
2. Bibimbap dressing
3. Blanched rice
4. Sliced carrots
5. Chopped green onions

Instructions

1. In a skillet, brown the ground meat.
2. Cook until the carrots are slightly softened in the skillet.
3. Stir together the bibimbap sauce and the meat and carrots.
4. Serve the Korean beef with boiled white rice.
5. Garnish with green onions, if desired.
6. Enjoy a tasty and speedy Korean beef bowl!

Primavera Pasta with Shrimp and Fresh Herbs

Ingredients

1. Pasta

2. Peeled and deveined shrimp

3. Tomatoes

4. Fresh basil

5. Extra virgin olive oil

Instructions

1. Cook the pasta as directed on the packet.

2. Sauté shrimp in olive oil in a skillet until done.

3. Cook until the halved cherry tomatoes are softened.

4. Toss together the cooked pasta, shrimp, and tomatoes.

5. Mix in the fresh basil.

6. Make a tasty pasta primavera with shrimp and fresh herbs!

Salmon with Teriyaki Glaze and Broccoli

Ingredients

1. Salmon fillets
2. Broccoli
3. Teriyaki marinade
4. Fresh garlic
5. Black sesame seed

Instructions

1. Preheat the oven to 400 °F (200°C).
2. Place the salmon on a baking sheet and surround it with the broccoli.
3. Brush fish with teriyaki sauce and minced garlic.
4. Bake for 12-15 minutes

5. Serve with broccoli and sesame seeds.

Skillet Cajun Chicken and Rice

Ingredients

1. Chicken thigh
2. Rice
3. Red bell peppers
4. Cajun spices
5. Chicken stock

Instructions

1. Cajun spice should be applied to chicken thighs.
2. Cook the chicken in a pan until it is browned.
3. Combine the rice, bell peppers, and chicken broth in a mixing bowl.
4. Simmer until the rice is soft and the chicken is done.

5. Cook yourself a tasty Cajun chicken and rice skillet!

Chickpea Curry (Vegan)

Ingredients

1. Chickpeas
2. Toasted tomatoes
3. Cocoa milk
4. Curry spice
5. Spinach

Instructions

1. Cook chickpeas in coconut milk in a saucepan.
2. Toss in the chopped tomatoes and curry powder.
3. Stir in the fresh spinach until it has wilted.
4. Make a simple and delicious vegetarian chickpea curry!

Grilled Lemon Herb Pork Chops

Ingredients

1. Pork loin chops
2. Lemon
3. Herb blend
4. Extra virgin olive oil
5. Fresh garlic

Instructions

1. Marinate pork chops in lemon juice, herbs, olive oil, and chopped garlic.
2. Grill until the meat is cooked through and the juices run clear.
3. Serve grilled lemon herb pork chops for a tasty meal!

Chapter 4

Snacks & Sides (To Get You Through the Day)

Chickpeas with Spices & Herbs, Roasted

Ingredients

1. Canned chickpeas
2. Extra virgin olive oil
3. Chilean paprika
4. Powdered garlic
5. Dried herbs (rosemary and thyme)

Instructions

1. Preheat the oven to 400 °F (200°C).
2. Drain and rinse canned chickpeas.
3. Combine chickpeas, olive oil, paprika, garlic powder, and dry herbs in a mixing bowl.

4. Distribute the chickpeas on a baking sheet.

5. Roast for 20-25 minutes, or until crispy, in a preheated oven.

6. Roasted chickpeas are a crispy and tasty snack!

Homemade Tortilla Chips with Guacamole

Ingredients

1. Avocados

2. Lemon juice

3. Red onion

4. Coriander

Instructions

1. In a mixing dish, combine avocados and lime juice.

2. Add the finely chopped red onion and cilantro and mix well.

3. Season to taste with salt and pepper.

4. Cut tortillas into triangles and bake until crispy for homemade tortilla chips.

5. Guacamole is a great snack when served with handmade tortilla chips.

Nachos with Apples, Yogurt, and Granola

Ingredients

1. Sliced apples

2. Greek yoghurt

3. Honey

4. Cereal

5. Cinnamon

Instructions

1. On a platter, arrange apple slices.

2. Drizzle the apple slices with Greek yogurt.

3. Drizzle with honey and top with granola.

4. For added taste, sprinkle with cinnamon.

5. Enjoy a platter of apple nachos that is both nutritious and filling!

Energy Bites with Peanut Butter and Banana

Ingredients

1. Nut butter

2. Rolled oatmeal

3. Honey

4. Mashed bananas

5. Chia seeds

Instructions

1. Combine peanut butter, rolled oats, honey, mashed bananas, and chia seeds in a mixing dish.

2. Chill the mixture for 30 minutes.

3. Roll into little energy bits.

4. Keep a few in the fridge for a fast and invigorating snack!

Eggs Hard-Boiled with Everything Bagel Seasoning

Ingredients

1. Eggs
2. Seasoning for everything bagel
3. Salt
4. Chili
5. Optional hot sauce

Instructions

1. Peel the eggs once they have been hard-boiled.
2. Season with everything bagel seasoning, salt, and pepper to taste.
3. Add a splash of spicy sauce for more heat if desired.

4. Hard-boiled eggs are a simple and protein-rich snack.

Bites of cucumber and hummus

Ingredients

1. Slice cucumber
2. Harissa
3. Tomatoes
4. Feta feta cheese
5. Olive oil

Instructions

1. Serve cucumber slices with hummus on the side.
2. Top each hummus-covered cucumber slice with a cherry tomato.
3. Garnish with feta cheese crumbles and olives.

4. Serve these cool Cucumber and Hummus Bites!

Chipotle Mayo Sweet Potato Wedges

Ingredients

1. Sugar potatoes
2. Extra virgin olive oil
3. Chipotle mayonnaise
4. Powdered garlic
5. Chilean paprika

Instructions

1. Preheat the oven to 400°F (200°C).
2. Sweet potatoes should be cut into wedges.
3. Toss the wedges in olive oil, garlic powder, and paprika to coat.
4. Bake until crispy, then serve with chipotle mayo.

5. Delicious Sweet Potato Wedges with Chipotle Mayo!

Fries with Baked Parmesan Zucchini

Ingredients

1. Zucchini
2. Parmiagano-Reggiano
3. Crusty bread
4. Powdered garlic
5. Italian seasoning

Instructions

1. Preheat the oven to 425°F (220°C).
2. Make zucchini fries out of it.
3. Combine the Parmesan, breadcrumbs, garlic powder, and Italian seasoning in a mixing bowl.

4. Bake until the zucchini fries are golden brown.

5. Serve with Baked Parmesan Zucchini Fries!

Cinnamon Chips with Fruit Salsa

Ingredients

1. Mixed fruits (strawberries, kiwi, pineapple e.t.c)
2. Cinnamon
3. Tortillas
4. Sugar
5. Lime

Instructions

1. Toss diced mixed fruits with cinnamon and sugar.
2. Separately, combine the sugar and cinnamon.

3. Cut the tortillas into chip shapes and top with the cinnamon-sugar mixture.

4. Bake until the bacon is crispy.

5. For a delicious and refreshing snack, pair the Fruit Salsa with Cinnamon Chips!

Chapter 5

Dessert (Sweet Finishes)

Ice Cream in a Chocolate Mug Cake

Ingredients

1. Whole wheat flour
2. Cocoa butter
3. Sugar
4. Milk
5. Vanilla flavouring

Instructions

1. Whisk together flour, cocoa powder, sugar, milk, and vanilla extract in a microwave-safe cup until smooth.
2. Microwave for 1-2 minutes on high, or until the cake is set.

3. Allow it to cool for a minute before topping
    with a scoop of your favorite ice cream.

4. Enjoy a simple and delicious chocolate
    cupcake!

Crispy Fruit Salad with Crumble Topping

Ingredients

1. Mixed fruits (berries and apples)

2. Oats

3. Dark brown sugar

4. Margarine

5. Cinnamon

Instructions

1. Preheat the oven to 350 °F (180°C).

2. In a baking dish, combine the fruits.

3. To prepare the crumble topping, combine oats, brown sugar, melted butter, and cinnamon in a mixing dish.

4. Crumble the topping over the mixed fruits.

5. Bake for 25-30 minutes, or until the fruit is bubbling and the topping is brown.

6. Make a warm and inviting fruit crisp!

Peanut Butter Cookies

Ingredients

1. Nut butter

2. Sugar

3. Eggs

Instructions

1. Preheat the oven to 350°F (180°C).

2. In a mixing dish, add peanut butter, sugar, and an egg.

3. Scoop out spoonfuls of the mixture onto a baking sheet.

4. To make a crosshatch design, flatten each biscuit using a fork.

5. Bake for 10-12 minutes, or until brown around the edges.

6. Enjoy these simple and tasty 3-ingredient peanut butter cookies!

Frozen Fruit and Yogurt Protein Shake

Ingredients

1. Protein shake

2. Frozen fruit (berries and bananas)

3. Greek yoghurt

4. Milk

Instructions

1. Blend protein powder, frozen fruit, Greek yogurt, and milk in a blender.
2. Blend until the mixture is smooth and creamy.
3. If necessary, add additional milk to get the desired consistency.
4. Sweeten with honey if desired.
5. Pour into a glass and enjoy a tasty protein shake!

Clusters of Dark Chocolate with Almond Bark

Ingredients

1. Chocolate, dark
2. Cashews
3. Fine sea salt
4. Optional dried fruit
5. Optional coconut flakes

Instructions

1. Melt the dark chocolate in the microwave or over the stovetop.
2. Stir in the almonds, sea salt, and any other ingredients if using.
3. Drop spoonfuls of the mixture onto a tray lined with parchment paper.
4. Place the clusters in the refrigerator to set.
5. Enjoy a delicious dark chocolate and almond treat by breaking it into pieces!

Cups of Strawberry Shortcake

Ingredients

1. Angel hair cake
2. Strawberry
3. Heavy whipping cream
4. Sugar
5. Vanilla flavour

Instructions

1. Make tiny cubes of angel food cake.
2. In cups, layer cake cubes with cut strawberries.
3. Finish with whipped cream and a dusting of sugar.
4. Drizzle with vanilla extract to taste.
5. Enjoy these delectable Strawberry Shortcake Cups!

Lemon Blueberry Pudding

Ingredients

1. Greek yoghurt
2. Strawberries
3. Lime curd
4. Cereal
5. Honey

Instructions

1. Layer Greek yogurt, blueberries, and lemon curd in a glass.

2. Rep the layers until the glass is filled.

3. Sprinkle with oats and sprinkle with honey.

4. Serve a delightful and refreshing Lemon Blueberry Parfait!

Macaroons with Coconut

Ingredients

1. Coconut shreds

2. Condensed sweetened milk

3. Vanilla flavor

4. Egg white

5. Chocolate pieces

Instructions

1. Preheat the oven to 325°F (163°C).

2. Combine the shredded coconut, sweetened condensed milk, vanilla essence, and egg whites in a mixing dish.

3. Place spoonfuls of the mixture on a baking sheet.

4. Bake till golden brown.

5. Melt chocolate chips and dip cooled macaroons in them.

6. Allow to set before serving these delicious Coconut Macaroons!

Bake-Free Energy Bites

Ingredients

1. Oats

2. Almond milk

3. Honey

4. Chocolate pieces

5. Chia seeds

Instructions

1. Combine oats, almond butter, honey, chocolate chips, and chia seeds in a mixing dish.
2. Chill the mixture for 30 minutes.
3. Roll into little energy bits.
4. Keep a few in the fridge for a fast and invigorating snack!

Bonus Section

Weekly Meal Prep Suggestions

Plan strategically

Spend some time at the start of the week planning your meals. To save time and money, look for items that may be used in numerous recipes.

Prep in Batches

Set aside time to prepare ingredients in batches. Prepare veggies, marinade meats, and prepare grains ahead of time to make it easier to put together meals throughout the week.

Storage Hacks

Properly keeping prepared items keeps them fresh and ready to use when you need them.

Grilling Instructions for Meat and Vegetables

Marinade Magic

Before grilling, marinate your meats to enhance their taste. Experiment with several marinades to find your favorite combinations.

Preheat for Success

Before you begin cooking, make sure your grill is warmed. This helps to sear the meat, seal in the juices, and create the perfect grill marks.

Grilled Veggies

Don't forget about the vegetables! Grilled vegetables with a drizzle of olive oil and herbs offer a tasty and healthful touch to your meals.

Spice Cabinet Essentials

Foundational Flavors

Start with the basics, such as salt, pepper, and garlic powder. These serve as the base for a variety of cuisines.

Bold choices

Experiment with stronger spices such as cumin, paprika, and Italian seasoning. These spices may bring depth and complexity to your cuisine.

Fresh Herb Burst

Keep a variety of fresh herbs on hand, such as basil, parsley, and cilantro. Just before serving, add them to your dishes for a blast of freshness.

Leftover Inspirations

Repurpose Leftovers Creatively:

Instead of viewing leftovers as a rerun, get creative with how you repurpose them. Make a fantastic chicken Caesar salad using leftover grilled chicken or a fast stir-fry with leftover vegetables.

Sandwich and Wrap Station

Set up a sandwich and wrap station stocked with a variety of spreads, cheeses, and sauces. It's a great way to turn boring leftovers into fascinating lunches.

Freeze for Later

If you have more leftovers than you can eat, try freezing them. You'll have quick and simple dinners for those days when you're pressed for time.

Other Resources for Busy Men

Meal Planning Tools: Look into online meal planning tools to assist you in properly schedule your weekly meals.

Cooking Apps: Get cooking apps that provide quick and easy recipes based on your tastes and dietary requirements.

Conclusion

Congratulations! You've reached the end of this 5-ingredient cookbook, and hopefully, the end of your culinary struggles. As you discovered, big flavor doesn't require a complicated kitchen dance. You've conquered hunger with minimal effort, proving that even the busiest man can feed himself delicious, satisfying meals.

But this book isn't just about quick fixes. It's about empowering you to take control of your kitchen and embrace the satisfaction of creating something nourishing for yourself. Remember, cooking can be an enjoyable adventure, not just a chore.

So, what's next? Keep exploring. Experiment with flavors, try new ingredients, and discover what truly fuels your inner beast. Remember, the possibilities are endless, and the kitchen is your playground.

Now go forth, conquer your hunger, and enjoy the journey!